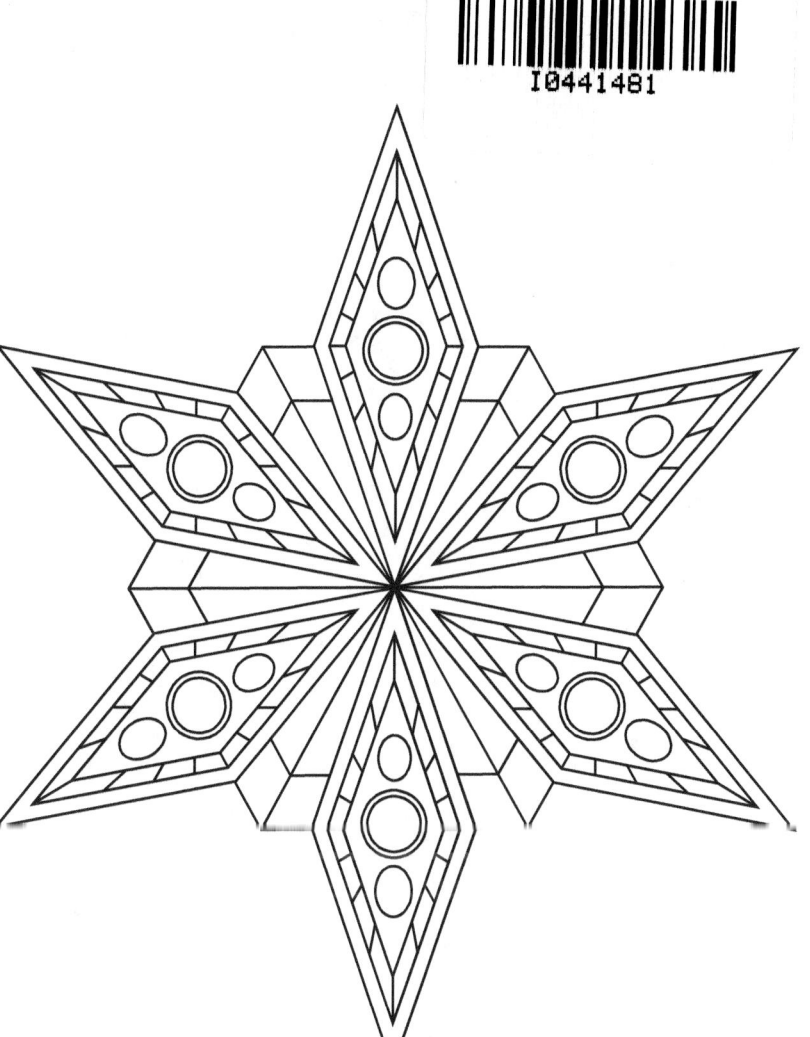

Colorist _____

Art by Tamara A. Cameron for *Mini Mandalas To Go!*
a ColorBinge Coloring Book for Adults
www.colorbinge.com

Welcome to the ColorBinge worldwide family! We would love to see your colored pages! Please join our private Facebook Group at https://www.facebook.com/groups/ColorBinge/ or just search for ColorBinge on Facebook.

You can find more about us and all the things we do at www.ColorBinge.com.

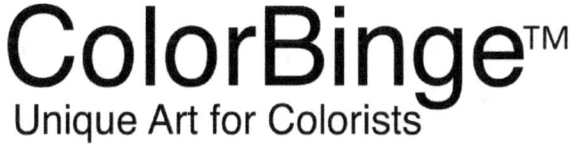

ColorBinge™
Unique Art for Colorists

We hope Mini Mandalas To Go brings you many relaxing and enjoyable hours of coloring!

# *Mini Mandalas To Go!*
## *A Relaxing Coloring Book for Busy Adults*

Coloring book & designs by
Tamara A. Cameron & Frank Plughoff

Pages at the end of this coloring book have intentionally
been left blank so colorists have a place to test out their
colors on this medium.

First Printing
2016

www.colorbinge.com

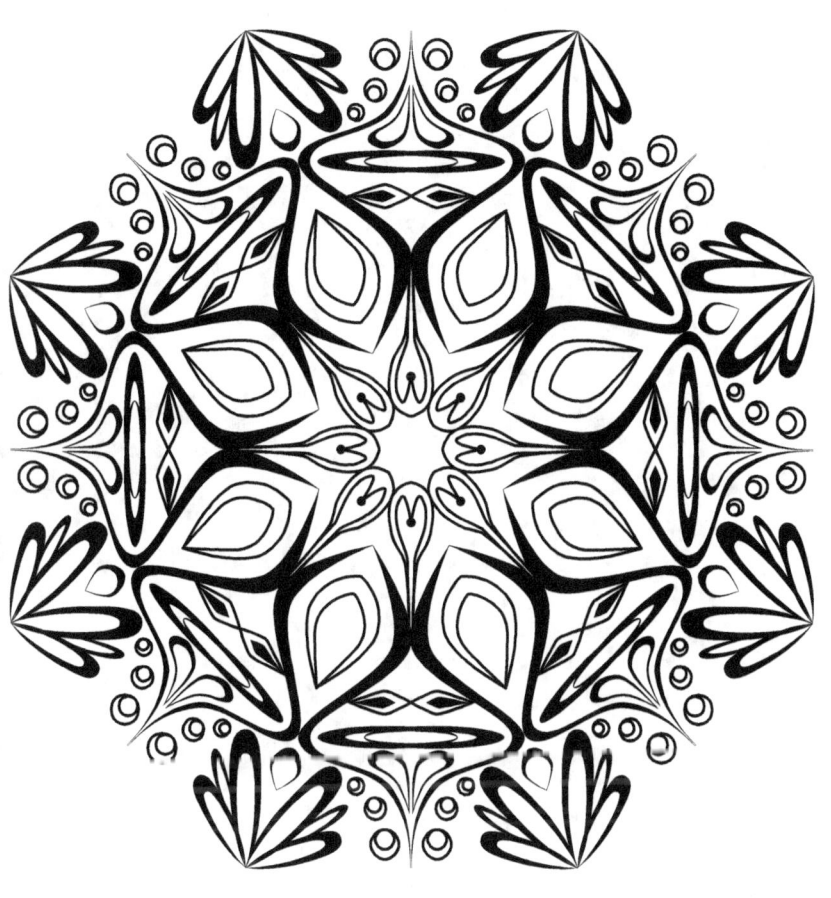

Colorist _____

Art by Frank Plughoff for *Mini Mandalas To Go!*

a ColorBinge Coloring Book for Adults

www.colorbinge.com

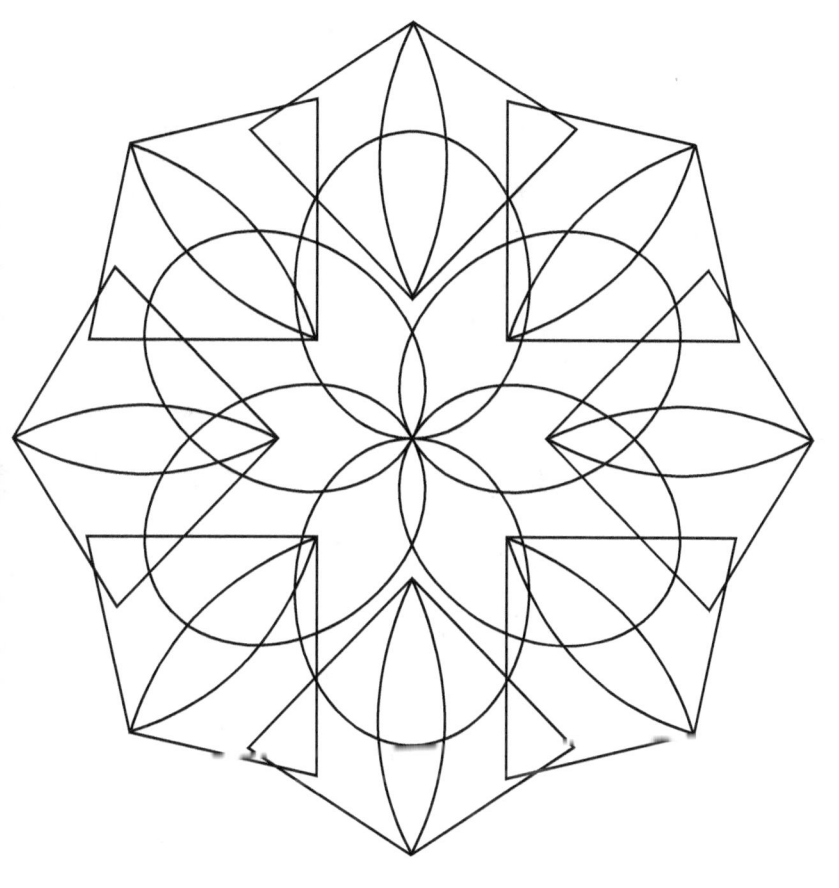

Colorist _____

Art by Tamara A. Cameron for *Mini Mandalas To Go!*
a ColorBinge Coloring Book for Adults
www.colorbinge.com

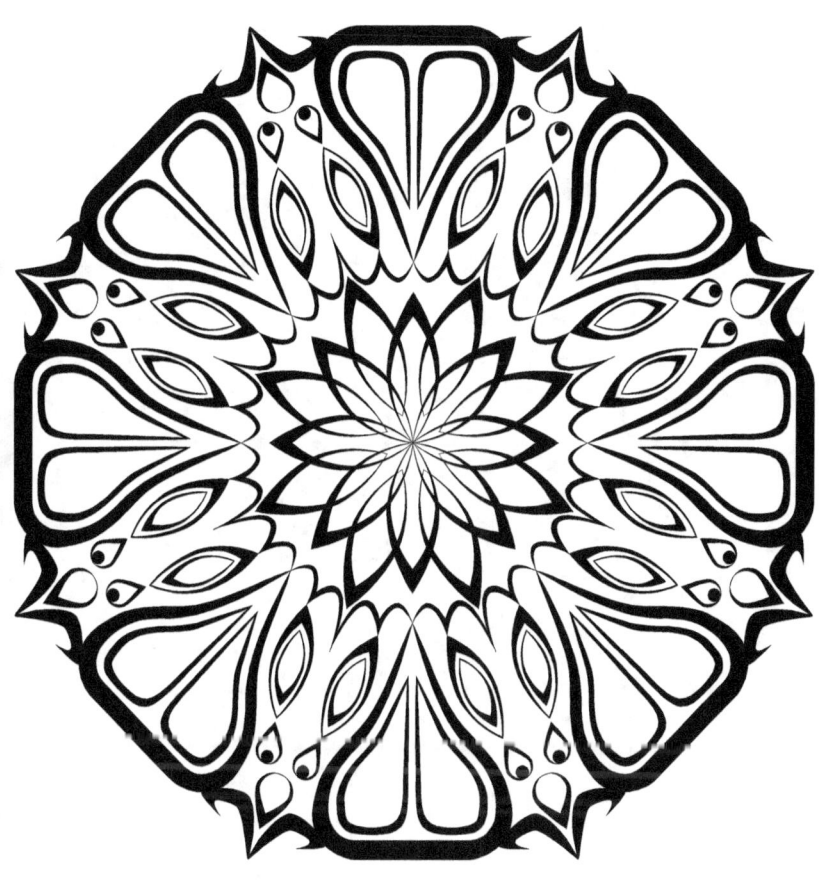

Colorist _____

Art by Frank Plughoff for *Mini Mandalas To Go!*
a ColorBinge Coloring Book for Adults
www.colorbinge.com

Colorist _____

Art by Tamara A. Cameron for *Mini Mandalas To Go!*
a ColorBinge Coloring Book for Adults
www.colorbinge.com

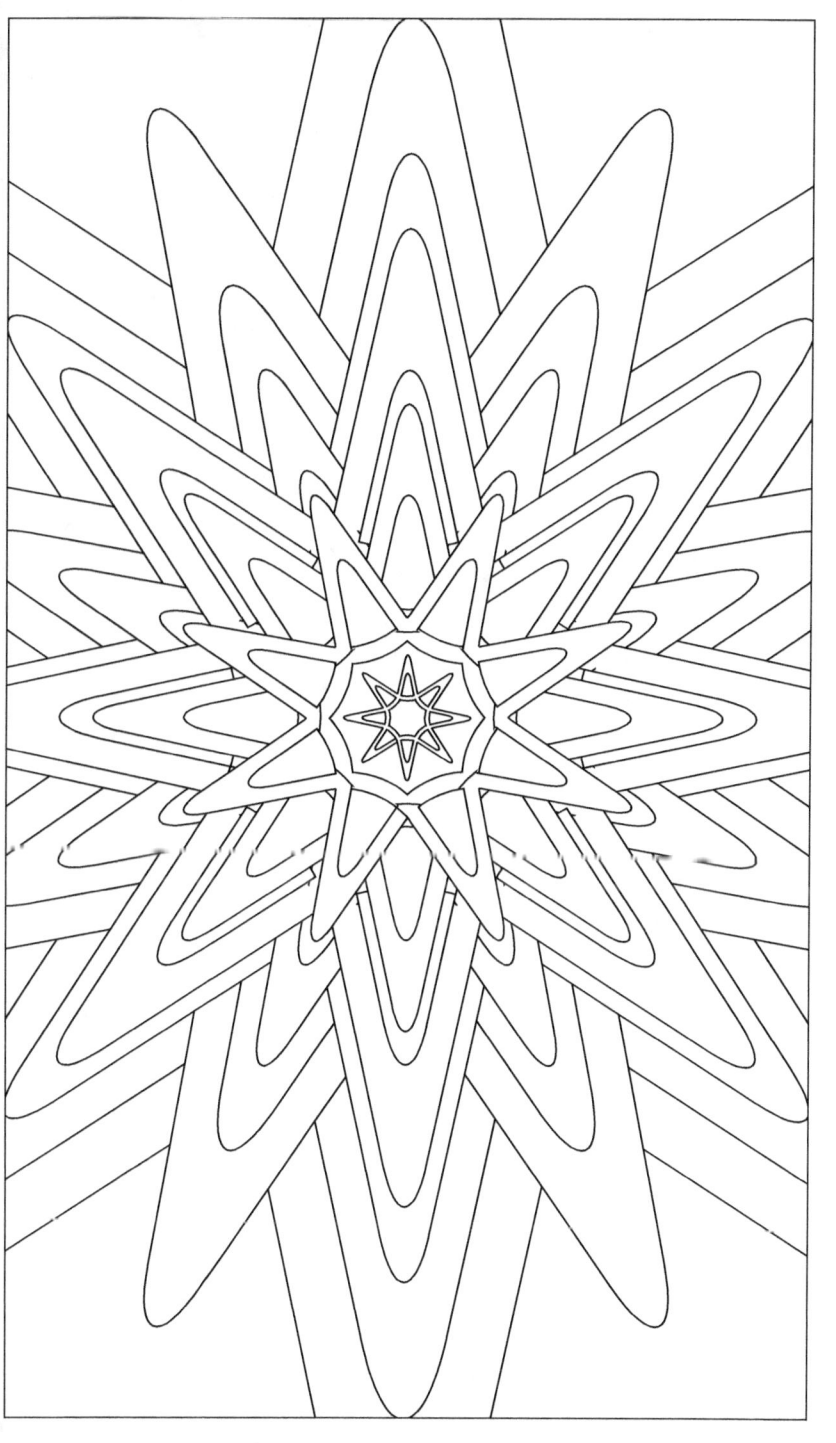

Colorist _____

Art by Frank Plughoff for *Mini Mandalas To Go!*
a ColorBinge Coloring Book for Adults
www.colorbinge.com

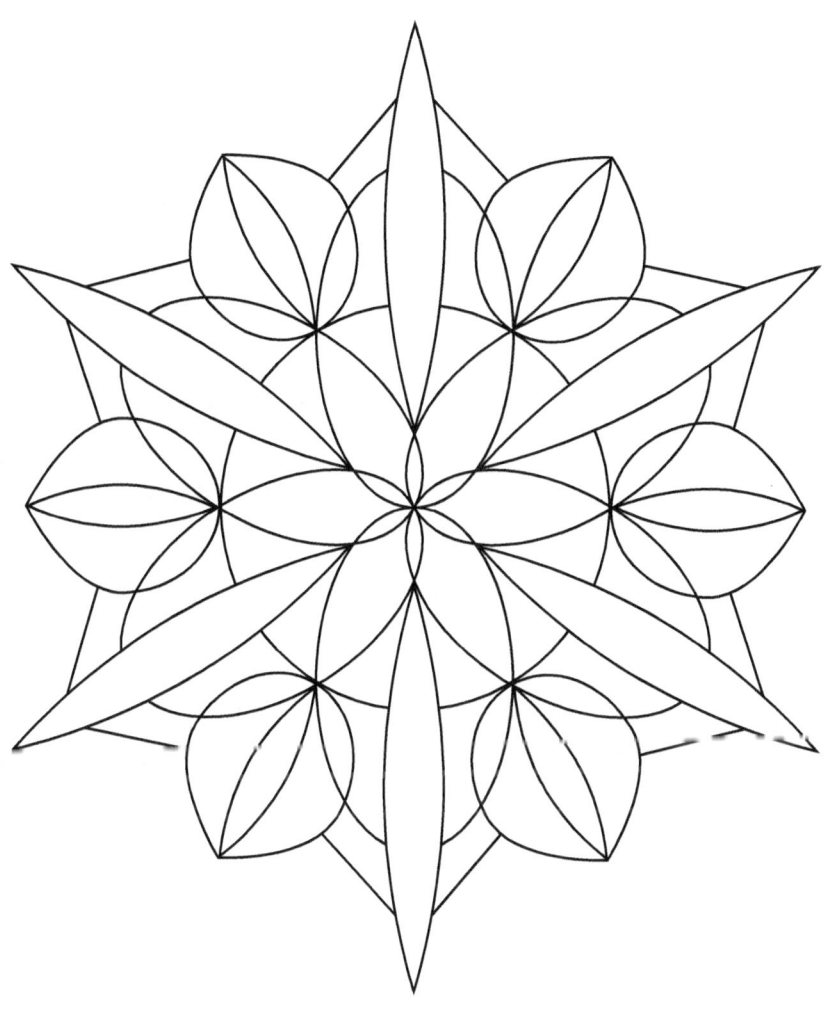

Colorist _____

Art by Tamara A. Cameron for *Mini Mandalas To Go!*
a ColorBinge Coloring Book for Adults
www.colorbinge.com

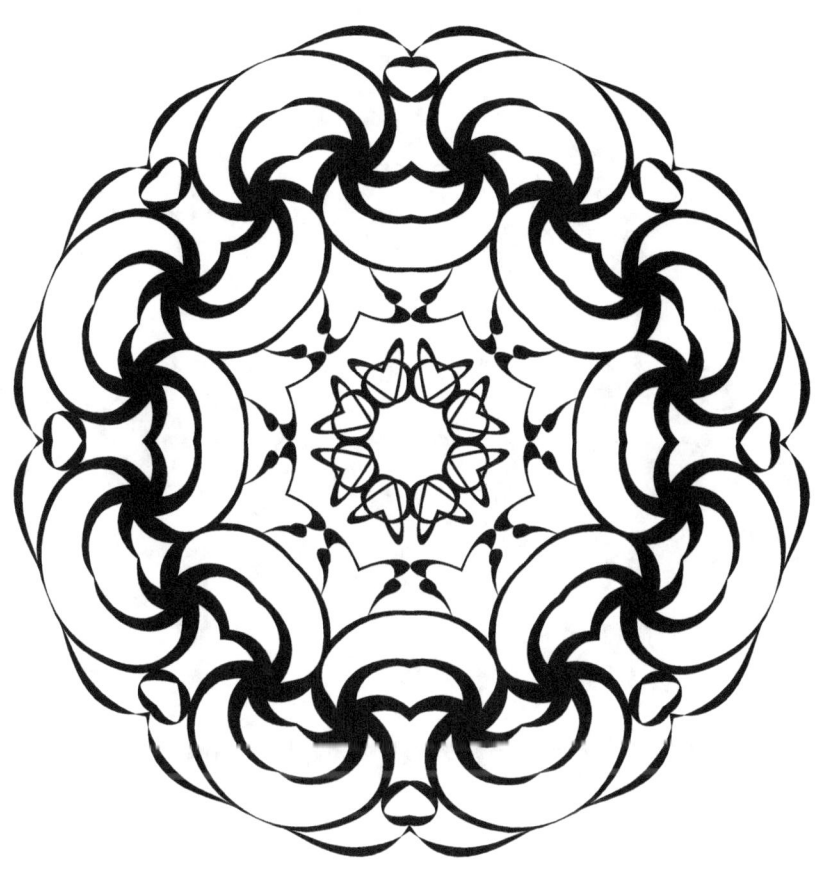

Colorist _____

Art by Frank Plughoff for *Mini Mandalas To Go!*
a ColorBinge Coloring Book for Adults
www.colorbinge.com

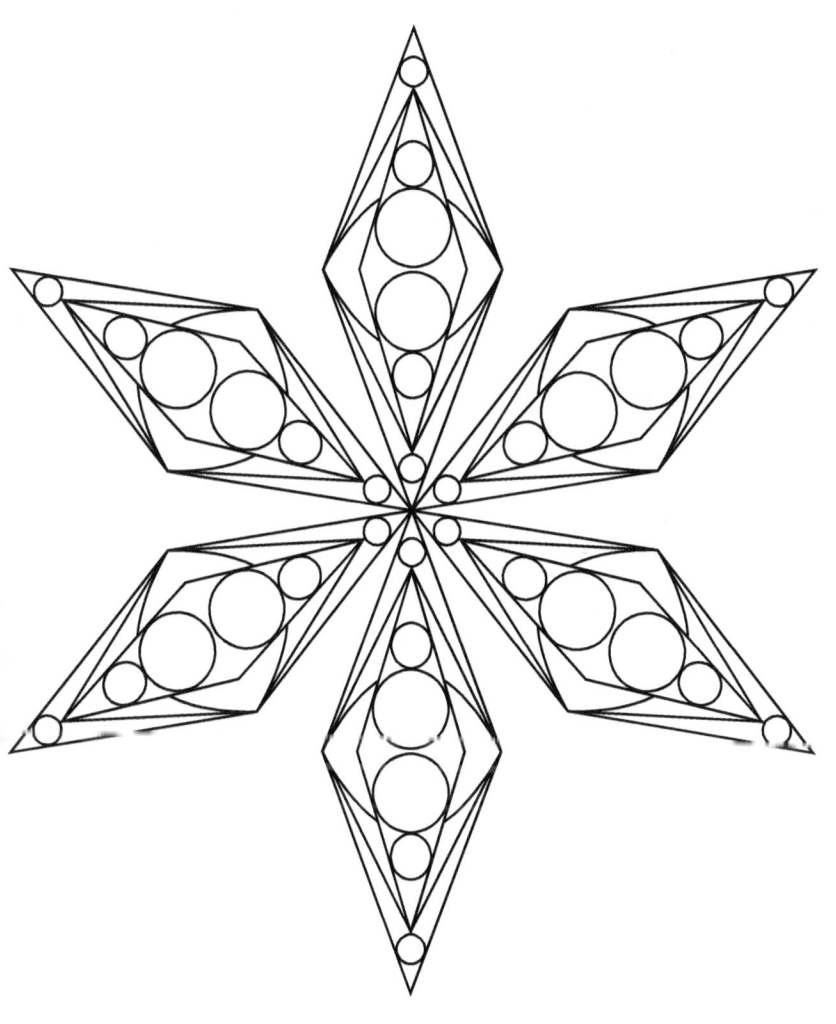

Colorist _____

Art by Tamara A. Cameron for *Mini Mandalas To Go!*
a ColorBinge Coloring Book for Adults
www.colorbinge.com

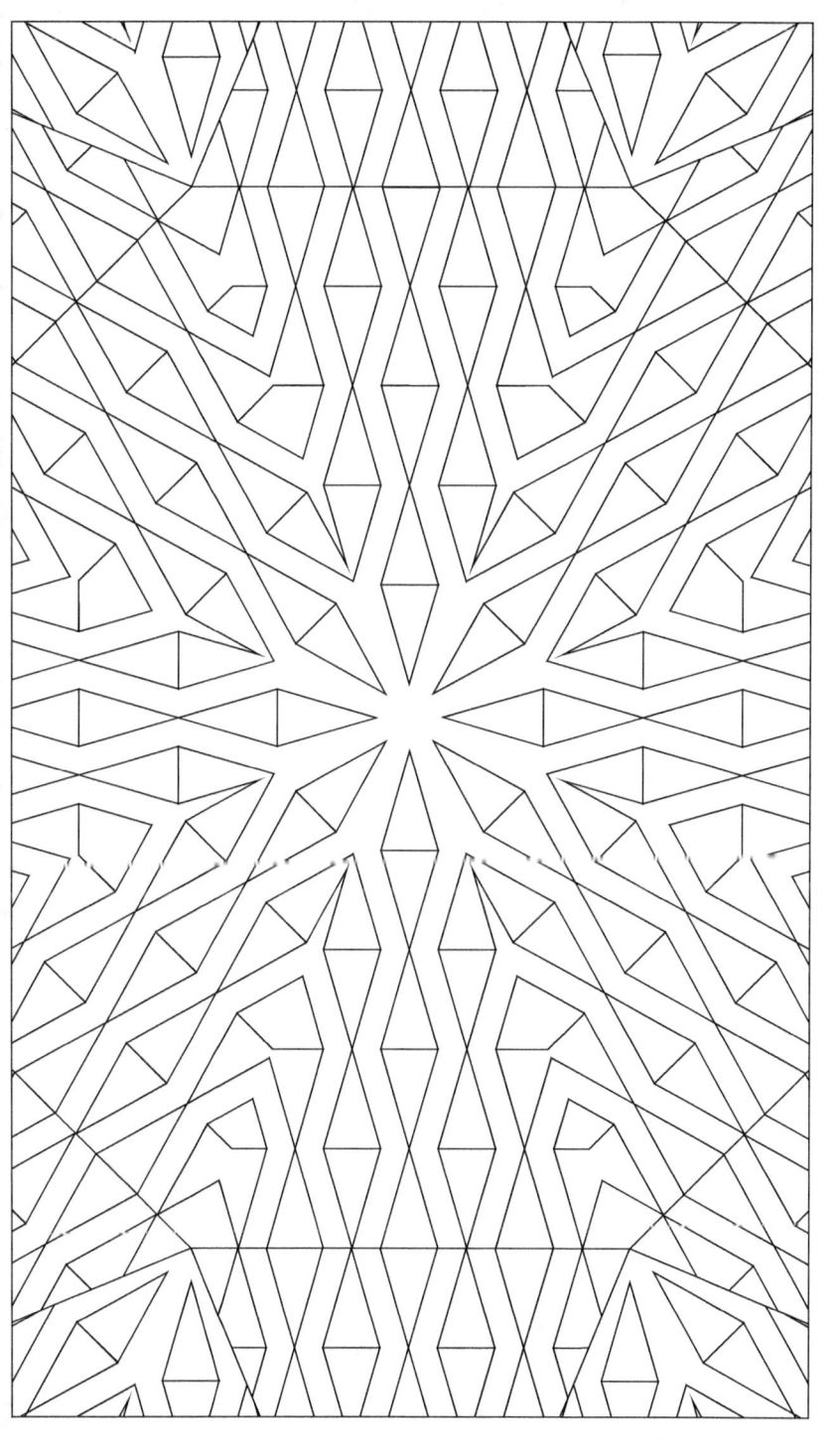

Colorist _____

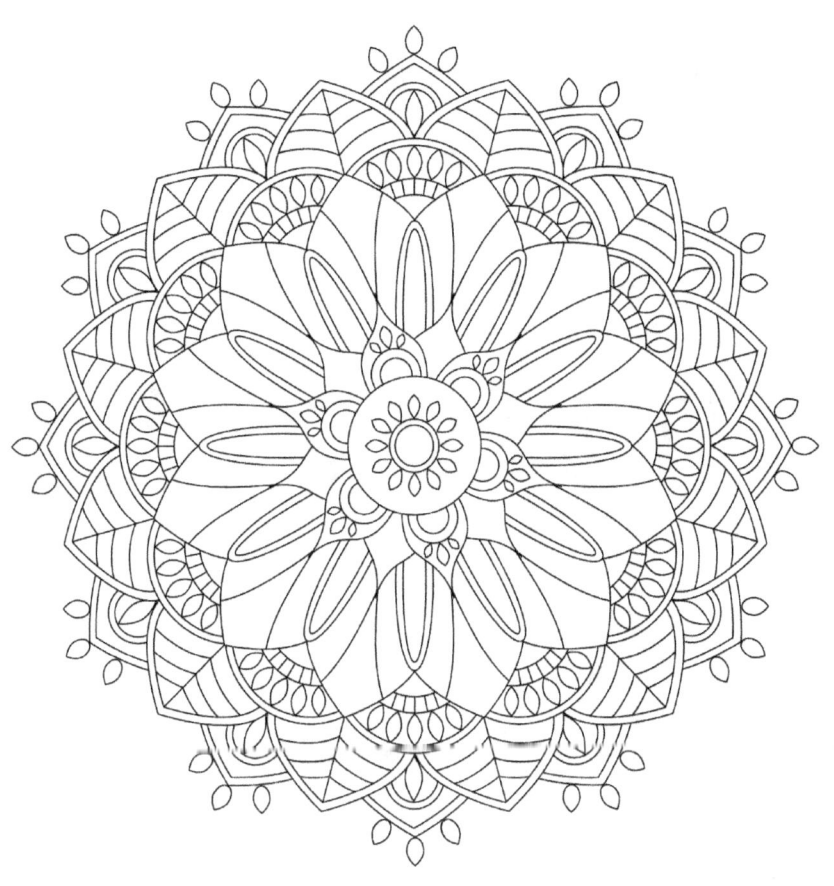

Colorist _____

Art by Tamara A. Cameron for *Mini Mandalas To Go!*
a ColorBinge Coloring Book for Adults
www.colorbinge.com

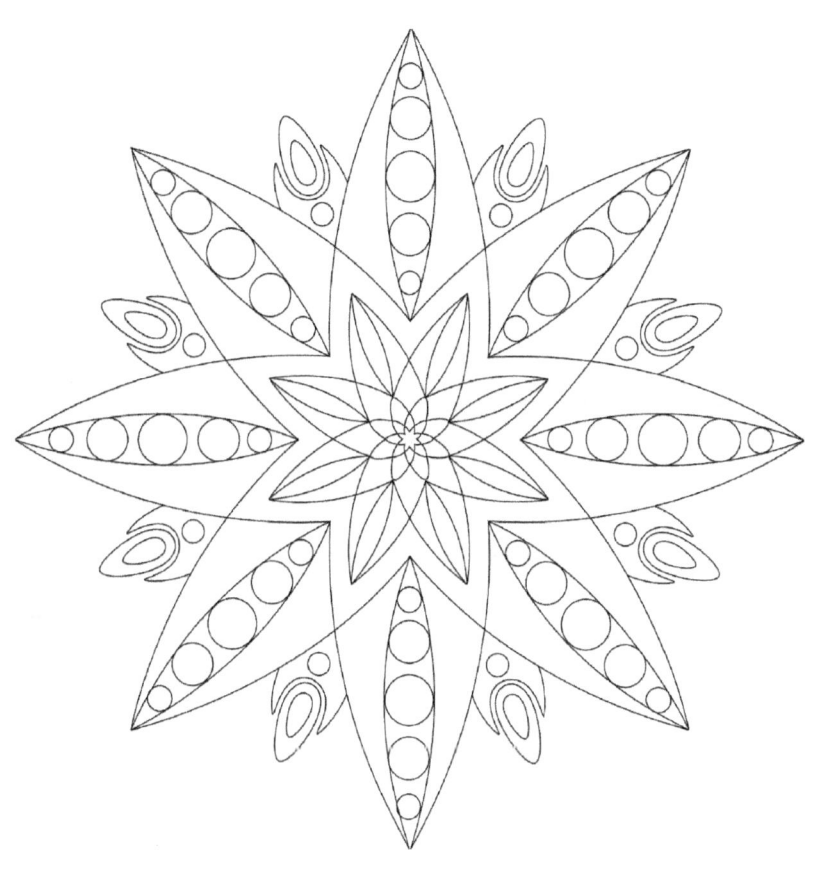

Colorist _____

Art by Frank Plughoff for *Mini Mandalas To Go!*
a ColorBinge Coloring Book for Adults
www.colorbinge.com

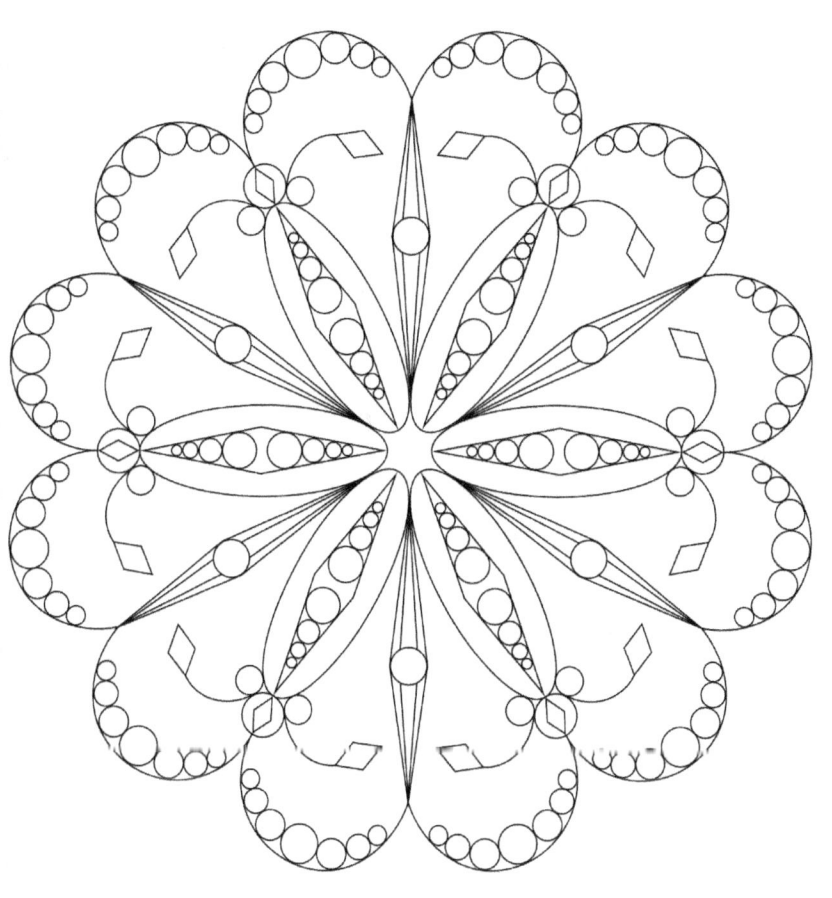

Colorist _____

Art by Tamara A. Cameron for *Mini Mandalas To Go!*
a ColorBinge Coloring Book for Adults
www.colorbinge.com

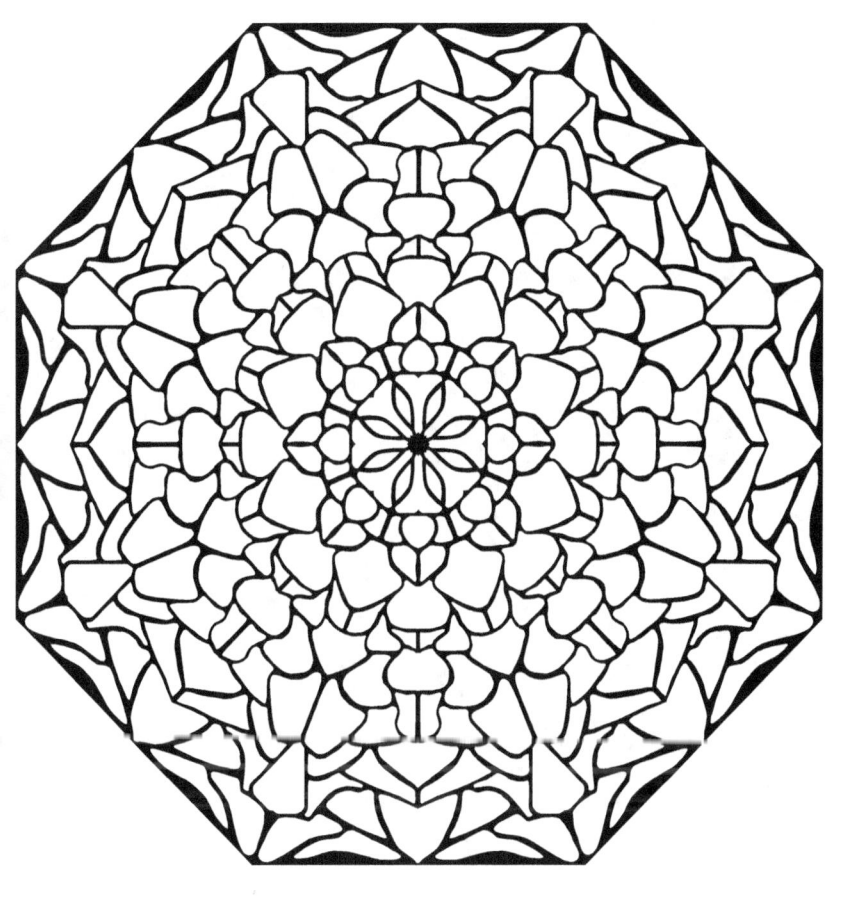

Colorist _____
Art by Frank Plughoff for *Mini Mandalas To Go!*
a ColorBinge Coloring Book for Adults
www.colorbinge.com

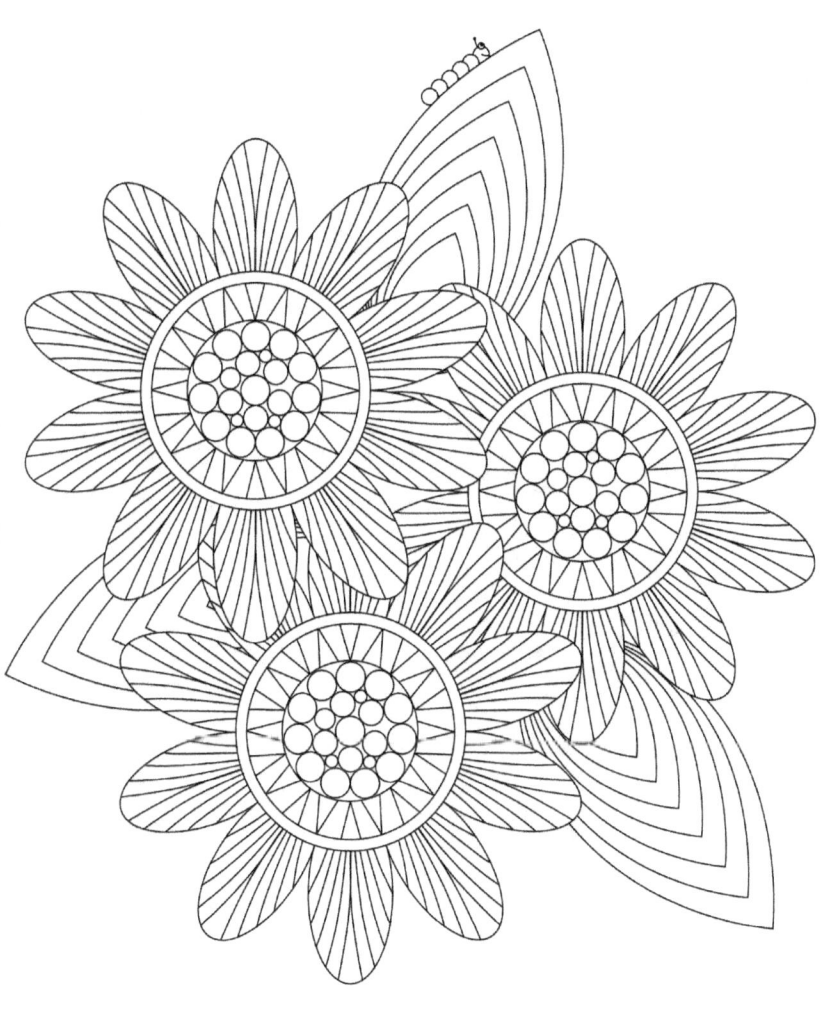

Colorist _____

Art by Tamara A. Cameron for *Mini Mandalas To Go!*
a ColorBinge Coloring Book for Adults
www.colorbinge.com

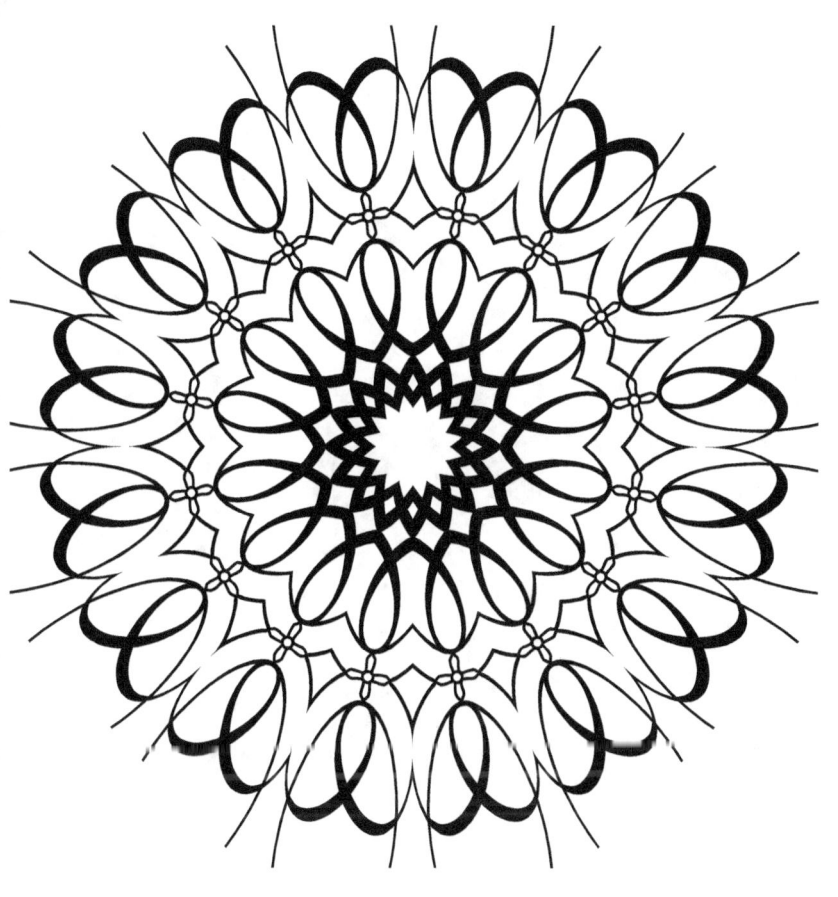

Colorist _____

Art by Frank Plughoff for *Mini Mandalas To Go!*
a ColorBinge Coloring Book for Adults
www.colorbinge.com

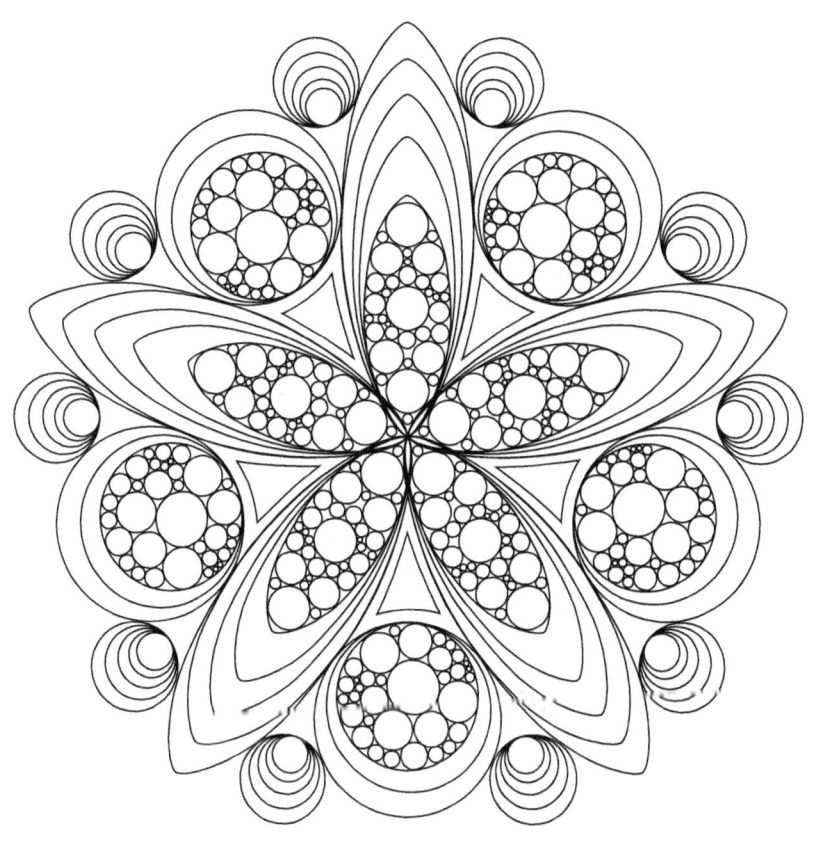

Colorist _____

Art by Tamara A. Cameron for *Mini Mandalas To Go!*

a ColorBinge Coloring Book for Adults

www.colorbinge.com

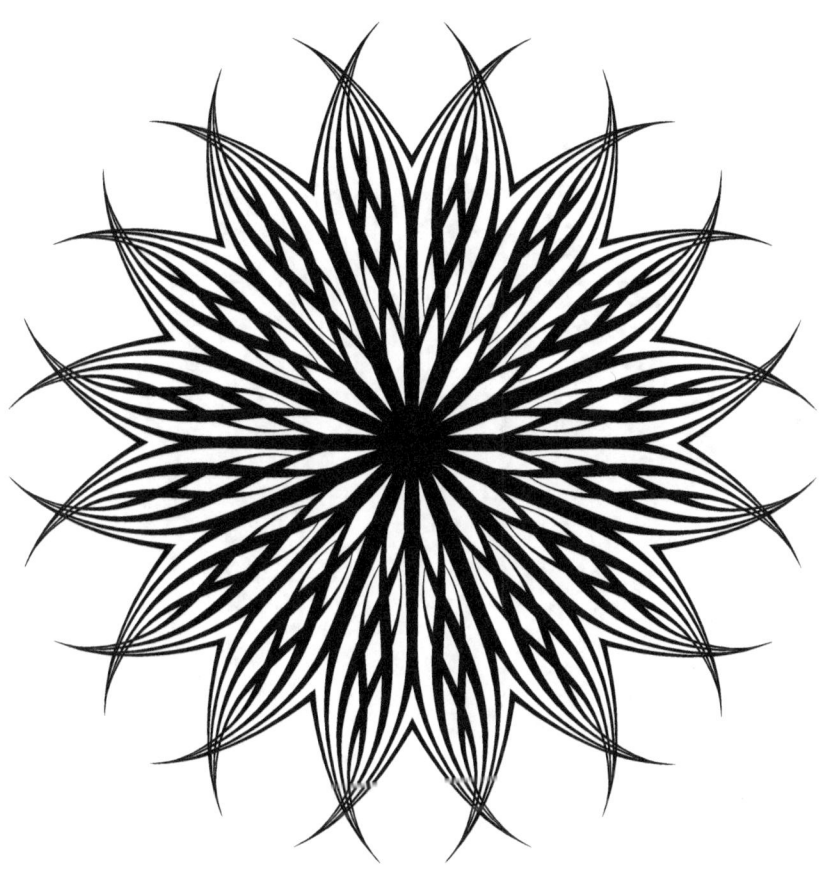

Colorist _____

Art by Frank Plughoff for **Mini Mandalas To Go!**
a ColorBinge Coloring Book for Adults
www.colorbinge.com

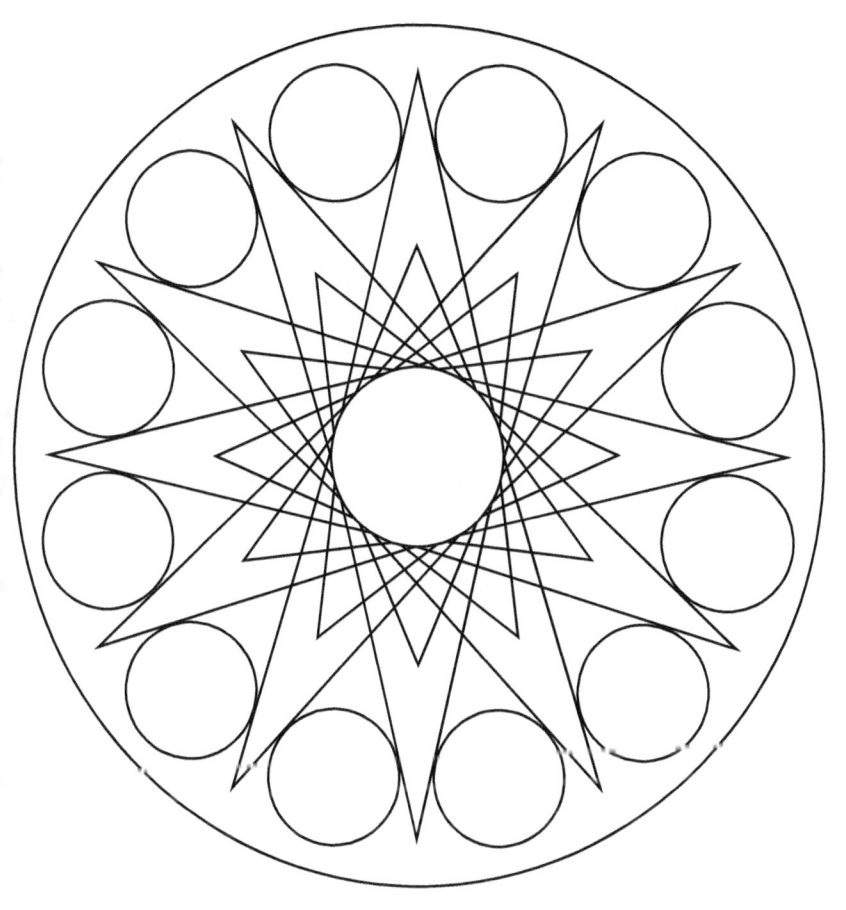

Colorist _____

Art by Tamara A. Cameron for *Mini Mandalas To Go!*
a ColorBinge Coloring Book for Adults
www.colorbinge.com

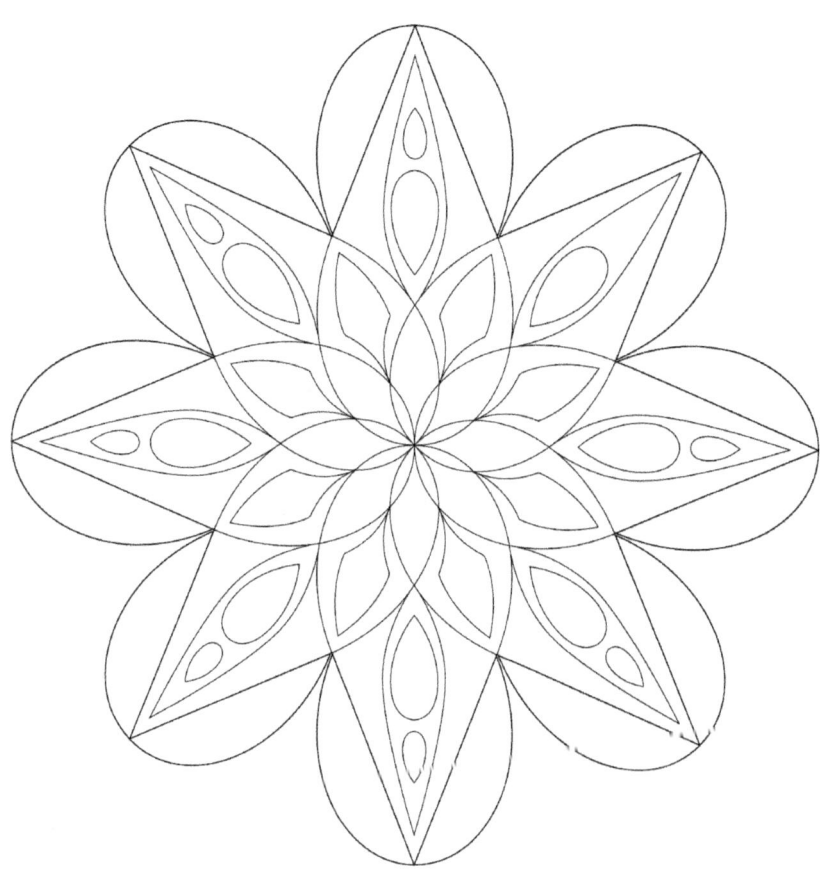

Colorist _____

Art by Frank Plughoff for *Mini Mandalas To Go!*
a ColorBinge Coloring Book for Adults
www.colorbinge.com

www.colorbinge.com
www.instagram.com/colorbinge/
https://www.etsy.com/shop/ColorBinge
www.facebook.com/groups/ColorBinge/

www.ingramcontent.com/pod-product-compliance
Lightning Source LLC
Chambersburg PA
CBHW070842310526
45793CB00011B/513